WOMEN IN THE GYM

How to Open and Operate a successful
Womans Only Fitness Facility

www.WomenintheGym.com
www.RebeccaFerente.com

By:Rebecca Ferente

Women in the Gym

Table of Contents

Meditation, Affirmation, Confirmation

I opened my first women-only outdoor boot camp in the spring of 2006. The park was dark and cold at 5 a.m. I started out with 3 clients I found from a newspaper ad I ran and grew to 50 clients within two months. I also expanded from one class time to two by adding a second class at 6 a.m.

I was a mom with a 13 year old, 3 year old, and a newborn at home. I worked two hours a day from 5 a.m. to 7 a.m. I never had to hire a babysitter or pay for daycare, and I made a 6 figure income.

More valuable than money were the wonderful ladies and the lives our little fitness community changed. We had working moms, stay-at-home moms, single girls, divorced women, lesbians, you name it. We welcomed everyone with open arms. Our community supported each other through divorces, surgeries, cancer, weddings, and graduations; and through it all, we grew and stayed together. Yes, people come and go. It's the ebb and flow of life, but most of my clients have stayed and formed lifelong bonds. My book is a journey, and your new niche business will be your destination.

I believe that one must "know thyself" before beginning a journey. Meditation, affirmations, and confidence are the three most important inner tools you will need to embark on your new journey. I'm sure you're thinking, "I just want to open a gym for women. What is she talking about?"

You must build a firm foundation within yourself before you embark on this journey. I understand that you want to open a business ASAP, but let's take a few moments and reflect on why you want to embark on this journey. I know you have seven days to complete my homework, and I hope you realize the firm foundation I'm giving to you.

Do you want to start a business to make money? Help others? Be popular? Because fitness is fun? Is this business about you, or is it about the clients you will be serving or both?

I would like to assign mental homework and give a task right out of the gate. Let's begin.

I want to start by defining meditation for you. **Meditation** is your ability to reach within your inner power and depth of your higher intelligence. I believe we use 10 percent of our brain power on a daily basis. We do mindless repetitive tasks, and the electronic world allows our brains to remain idle most of the time. When you meditate, you are tapping into the depths of your brain, searching and rescuing the deep answers to all your questions, and finding solutions to meet your needs. Meditation is not something you do for one week and then never revisit the task. Meditation needs to be performed daily. You have all the answers to your life's questions. It's up to you to tap into that energy and use it to be amazing in business and in life.

HOMEWORK #1 (Complete on Days 1 & 4)

Grab a sheet of paper and write down 15 reasons you want to start a fitness business that serves a WOMEN ONLY client base. Great job! You gave me 20 reasons instead of 15! Wow! Your enthusiasm is awesome! Now, I want you to put that paper out of sight. During Days 1, 2, and 3, I want you to find a quiet place with no distractions, find a timer, and set it for 12 minutes. Practice this exercise twice a day. The best times would be when you first wake up and at the end of the day. Now take a deep breath to fill your lungs up with air and breathe out. I want you to repeat this breathing exercise for the entire 12 minutes. Clear your mind, and DO NOT FORCE thoughts to come in. Relax and let your inner voice take over. If something negative comes in to your train of thought, promptly tell it "no thank you, not now" and resume focusing on your breathing and allow positive thoughts to flow.

Welcome to Day 4. Today, I would like you to grab a fresh sheet of paper and write down 10 reasons you want to start a fitness business that serves WOMEN ONLY. Now place that sheet of paper out of sight.

Meditation and affirmations go hand in hand. **Affirmations** are defined as power thoughts that will change your life. Your mind is a powerful tool. When you say something, it is true in your world. In order to make an affirmation a reality, you need to repeat it throughout the day and truly believe it. Affirmations are not wishes or hopes. Affirmations are truths that lead us to our goals.

My favorite affirmations are:

- My cash flow is constantly increasing.

- Clients are seeking us.

- I refuse to allow chaos in my life!

- Today is an awesome day.

On Days 4, 5, 6, and 7, continue to meditate. In order to form your own powerful life, focus on your meditations. I encourage you to start a meditation journal to reflect on the clear messages received. At the end of your sessions, write down your inspirational thoughts. Review your journal often and use those messages to form daily inspiring affirmations.

Another way to form inspiring affirmations is to write down your personal goals. Grab a sheet of paper, and at the top write the words "Happiness," "Prosperity," and "Tasks." Under each, define what that word means to you.

Just because you say an affirmation once, it will not become a truth or reality. What we concentrate on increases. The first time you say an affirmation, think of it as a tear drop on your desk. The more you reflect on your affirmation each day, the small drop will expand to a puddle, then a river, and before you know it, an ocean, and eventually your affirmation will be real! Our spoken words become real when we believe them and act upon them.

HOMEWORK #2

Do not start this task until seven full days of meditation have occurred.

Retrieve your sheets of paper from HOMEWORK #1, and grab your meditation journal and your personal goal sheets.

Spread all your papers out on the surface in front of you. You should have 25 reasons to open a women's only gym, a collection of key thoughts from your daily meditations, and two to five affirmations. Grab a new sheet of paper after reflecting on your data and write five reasons to open a women only gym and two affirmations. Place the sheet with the five reasons to open a women's only gym at the top of your stack of papers and file it for now. Now, we need to make our affirmations a reality.

If you have a wireless device that will notify you daily, please type your affirmations into the calendar and schedule them to appear on your phone twice a day at times you will be able to focus and reflect when they appear on your screen. If technology is not at your fingertips, grab a sheet of paper and write your affirmation down and post it at your desk, next to your bed, or anywhere you reside part of the day.

All that's left to "know thyself" is confidence. **Confidence** is two fold. It's found inside and shown outside of every human being. We will begin with "inside." Meditation and affirmations will help you build confidence within. As we continue building our foundation for success, we must be strong enough to handle the lowest of lows on our journey to success in business and life. Let me tell you from my own firsthand experience: this journey will not be easy, and you will have many days and nights feeling alone and struggling to make your new business a success. During these times you will need to reflect and go within yourself utilizing your meditation and affirmations to maintain your confidence, reflect upon your goals, and move forward.

Confidence on the outside starts with something as simple as pulling your shoulders back and down, look people in the eye, shake hands with those you meet, and listen to what others have to say. Your demeanor and body language will reflect your true confidence, and people will be attracted to you.

Are you ready to become a successful entrepreneur in the women's only market? If you're reading my book in search of a safe, EASY, fast way to open a business, close my book right now! This journey will be the hardest up-and-down rollercoaster ride of your life! Heed my warning: this journey is not for the weak. Some months you will make thousands of dollars, and others you will not make one dollar. If you like the security of a regular bi-weekly pay check, close my book NOW! Clients behave like children at times, and you will be required to go as far as firing clients if they hurt your business. Can you handle that? You already have bills from home, and now you will have bills from your business. You will pay rents, mortgages, power bills, phone bills, etc. If the AC breaks at your gym, the landlord does not repair it -- you do. How will you pay for it?

On the flip side, if you're tired of watching life pass you by and you're ready to take a risk and jump in with two feet, you will be rewarded. The freedom to own your own business is amazing. Getting up each day and helping like-minded individuals get in shape and improve their lifestyle is the best job ever. Setting your own hours and having time to pick up the kids from school are priceless. Finding prosperity doing what you love is an incredible reward. You will experience the highest of the highs and the lowest of the lows, but you report to yourself. You must give 110% to make a successful business.

Go confidently in the direction of your dreams! **Live the life** you've imagined.
- Thoreau

Niche Market

If the first paragraph left a pit in your stomach and you're now having second thoughts, re-read chapter one and do the homework again. If you're even more excited and ready for the most rewarding challenge of your life, let's get this business STARTED!

We have defined our market as women only. When you narrow your market down to a niche, you soon come to realize that it's easier to focus on a business plan. Yes, I said it -- business plan. I don't encourage you to overwhelm yourself writing one, but you do need a map to take you on the journey.

A basic business plan will define your market and help you stay focused on that market. Templates are available on the web. Do not let this task overwhelm you. Business plans can change year to year, so do not stress over this task.

If you're applying for a loan or looking for investors, your business plan becomes even more important and will determine the amount of investment funds received. A local SCORE association can guide you when writing this type of business plan, and several online resources are available at your fingertips.

I opened my first women only fitness business in 2006. I opened it during the boom of outdoor boot camps, and I quickly realized they were made up of 90% women. As I looked at my client base, a light bulb went off. I decided to change my business plan and focus 100% on the needs of MYSELF. Yes, I said it -- be selfish and focus on yourself. You are your own BEST CLIENT. If you like it, the clients you attract will as well. Female owners in the women's only market make a ton of cash and have a huge client base, because they set up their business model around their own wants and needs. I highly suggest gathering an all-female round table of 3-4 different family/friends to get the ladies' perspective on your facilities' offerings.

Research has shown that women are spending billions of dollars each year on fitness and nutrition, and now is the time to tap into that market.

For example, if you love to lift weights, buy bars and bumpers designed for women and our small features, a.k.a. skinny bars and light bumpers. If endurance is your thing, buy jump ropes if you were once that little girl at recess pulling out the jump rope from the toy bucket spending your time jumping rope with your girlfriends. As a woman, you deal with monthly hormonal changes. As we age, menopause comes into play. Who better than fellow women to guide ladies through nutrition and body changes?

Nutrition is 85% of the overall health equation. Don't skimp on nutrition guidance. If you're not certified or do not have nutritional education, I strongly suggest educating yourself ASAP! Women, more than ever, need your help. It is my belief that you are what you eat, and the key to a healthy body is what we put in it. Women struggle with weight and body image issues, and your support is needed more than ever. You have many options regarding weight loss support and maintenance for your clients. You can hire a certified nutritionist or co-market with one. Guide your clients to your favorite weight loss website or tools. Have fitness challenges in your gym. Just remember that one diet does not fit all, and each client is an individual. I personally recommend sitting down with each client and asking them to complete a goal sheet. Not every client is interested in nutrition. Many are visiting you to work out only. For the clients that are looking for your help in the weight loss department, offer grocery store tours, online education referrals, and direct referrals to a nutrition specialist.

Women struggle with bone loss, puffy tummies, and saggy boobs thanks to childbirth and aging. Strong is the new sexy at any age!

You will quickly realize many benefits to opening a women's only facility. First off is cost of equipment. Many items are sold by the pound. If you are opening a gym that offers a weight lifting program, which is needed by all females at least 3 times per week, you can purchase lighter barbells and weights and save a ton of money. Kettle bells are sold per weight as well as medicine balls, just to name a few items. Thousands of dollars are saved versus opening up a co-ed facility.

The difference between men and women when it comes to fitness is, in a nutshell: men jump in and try everything with no regard for safety, and women tend to think twice and worry about "breaking a leg." Be prepared to modify movements and dish out a lot of support and reinforcement to your girls. They can do it, and they will surprise themselves. But this will take time and patience from the coaching department. After you have been in business for a few months, you may choose to offer classes with varied levels so you do not hold anyone back, yet you still need to make everyone feel important and valued.

I would like to break down female clients by age group. **Twenty something's** may be fast and strong, still in college, or just graduated with the freshman 15 to lose. They are very self conscious and may be looking for a mate -- but not in the gym. In the gym, they want to let their hair down and look a mess while getting fit. This age group will also look up to you. They are very fast learners who tend to listen to your fitness cues well.

Thirty something's may have just had a child or still have the weight on them from past pregnancies. Many thirty-something's are busy, single, working women. They have one hour to give you and want to get in and out before their next task. This group listens well, but in all honestly, they tend to have their mind on something else. You will need to watch them closely, because they can lift heavy and run the fastest -- but they are the most prone group to injuries.

Forty something's just turned a biological corner, and everything they eat sticks to their thighs and guts. They have to work twice as hard to lose weight, and, due to hormonal changes, may have a weaker bone structure. It's very important to have this group stretch and see a doctor/chiropractor regularly to improve their body flexibility in order to be able to workout regularly without nagging injuries.

Fifty something's are a very respectful, happy-to-be-in-the-gym community. They come for light weightlifting to improve bone density and enjoy being in a group with both younger and older women. In my opinion, they inspire the group the most.

Sixty and seventy something's are AWESOME! They have aches and pains, yet they push through the pain. Most will tell you they wake up sore every morning, and the more they move throughout the day, the better they feel. They tend to prefer to pay annually, rather than monthly. They are committed and very much appreciate all you do in the modification of skills to allow them to be in class with everyone.

In our female niche market, you will need to emphasize quality, building personal connections with your clients, and offering outstanding customer service. If you're going into business with the sole purpose of making money, you more than likely will not. If you're trying to make a difference in people's lives, you'll find true success. Build a "community" from Day 1 with your girls.

"Serve a Million People and Make a Million Dollars."

Exploring the Marketing World

Local Newspaper and TV

More than likely, your facility will be a one-of-a-kind "women's only facility" in your community. That is a story in itself. Make the call and convey how exciting this is for your community. A newspaper article will bring in more clients than an ad. Please be sure to have a great story to tell; it should be all about "you," because you're your own BEST client. Typically, morning TV shows love to do segments with a workout so grab your best friends and put on a great show with lots of smiles and laughter.

Flyers

This type of door-to-door marketing is cost saving. Typically, a flyer company will charge 7-10 cents per paper. To save even more money, print your own flyers and just ask the flyer company to deliver.

Online

Google ads will place you at the top of the search results, and Facebook has recently become very popular. Each week, I take a photo of my clients working out in the gym and pay a small fee to "boost" the post to my members' friends; this has really paid off and become a super cheap marketing tool that brings in 2-3 new people each week.

Cross Market

Approach other businesses that your client base will use in conjunction with your establishment. For example, we work with a local hot yoga studio and have Wednesday night stretch classes. I also encourage you to entertain the idea of welcoming other like-minded female-based businesses in your space to set up permanent offices or specific day/ time visits with them. These include female massage therapists, physical therapists, and demagogical professionals, to name a few.

Ambassador Program

Each month, spotlight a business in your community. Have a representative from that business come in and work out with your community. At the end of the workout, the ambassador can hand out samples or do a demo of their product. It's great for your community and a fantastic cross-marketing promotion, because you will both market your business to each other's clients and friends. I highly encourage you to use the Facebook platform for this.

Co-Advertising

Use this tool with another female-based business. For example, we have sent out flyers with a local female real-estate agent. Her ad is on the front of the flyer, and ours is on the back. It's win-win for both of us and a 50% cost savings as well.

Join the local Chamber of Commerce

Offer FREE gifts to local women's clubs. Most of these clubs have meetings and give away door prizes. A few free visits to the gym will go a long way.

Personally, I believe you will get the most bang for your buck taking advantage of the digital age in which we live. The business WEB SITE and FACEBOOK page will be the first points of contact with potential clients. Spend money on your web site and make sure it looks great on both the computer screen and on a cell phone. You will find many templates to build your own web site, but I suggest shopping around for an affordable web site designer. These professionals know how to place key words on your website which will place your business at the top of search engines. And let's not forget Facebook -- who doesn't have a Facebook account? People share pictures and talk about their daily lives. YOUR BUSINESS needs to be a part of their lives. In addition to people talking to their friends about your gym, you will post daily photos of the girls working out. Most women are very visual, and viewing their friends' smiling while losing weight and lifting heavy stuff is the best marketing you will ever have.

The cost to advertise on Facebook was $10. I posted the photo on the gym's Facebook page and wrote a call to action tag line above it. When you "boost" a page, you can start out as low as $5.00. And as more people see your post, you can add money and pay as you go based on the reply. Facebook boosting gives you the option to send it out to your friends and your friends' "friends" or to choose local zip codes and encourage new clientele to join.

Your new gym community will become your best marketing tool. Once you have established a community, you will find that you no longer need to pay for advertising. If you offer incredible coaching and a fun atmosphere, your clients will take over and market for you. Ladies love to buy clothing. Make sure your rack is stocked with T-Shirts and tanks with a fun saying and your GYM LOGO. Clients will wear these proudly around town and tell their friends to join. Offer your clients rewards for bringing in their friends. For example, we give members $10 off their monthly membership fee for every client they bring in who joins the gym. Ladies night out, book clubs, business meet-ups, group fitness adventures on weekends like hiking, biking, etc are additional ways to build your community.

Marketing to women only will be very easy if you're the only one in town operating a gender specific gym. Take out an ad and invite the ladies. Encourage them to bring their friends and daughters. I have found, in addition to my female-based programming, that our community of like-minded girls really looks forward to spending an hour together working out each day. They don't have to worry about putting on makeup. The girls tend to feel less self-conscious, and the atmosphere has a competitive, but fun, tone to it.

How to.........

We have focused on "you" and your new niche market. Now it's time to focus on the HOW TO OPEN A BUSINESS side of this equation.

Let's start with asking if this will be a sole proprietorship or if it will have multiple owners. I strongly encourage you to consult a professional attorney or tax accountant for guidance in this important decision. There are benefits to both scenarios. If you're in business with yourself, you're in control; and for many of us, that's the way to go. At the end of the day if things are going great, you pat yourself on the back and celebrate your success. If you have hit a rough patch, you have no one to blame but yourself. As the saying goes, it's lonely at the top; but I would rather be at the top alone than at the top fighting with a friend!

That brings us into partnerships. I do not recommend going into business with your best friend or a family member unless they are "investors only." Owning a business is tough, and getting a business off the ground that has zero clients is even harder. If your friend is used to a weekly paycheck and thrives on security, DO NOT GO INTO BUSINESS with them. If you do choose to go into business with a friend, consult an attorney and write up a partnership agreement ASAP before you spend a dime on opening the gym!

I feel the need to scare you out of a partnership with friends or family, so let's review a few scenarios. You decide you cannot open this venture without your workout pal Maggie. Maggie is a stay-at-home mom, and her husband is an executive. They have a few dollars saved, and Maggie has convinced her hubby that this is an awesome investment. He takes a loan from his 401k and gives it to Maggie, who has never worked outside the home and always had her needs met by her husband. You apply for a business license, skip the partnership agreement, and start shopping for a space and equipment. What girl does not like to shop! An affordable location is found. You debate about a three or five year lease, and Maggie's husband steps in and kindly forces you to sign a three year lease with larger rent payments. No big deal this time – "he was probably correct," you say to yourself and move on. You grab the equipment list and start shopping online. You're a true bargain hunter at heart but understand you need commercial quality. Maggie and her husband flip out when they see how much you have spent. After a three hour meeting regarding the budget, you win this battle. Currently, we are 1-1 in battles won/lost.

It's grand opening day, and all parties think they made it and that a ton of clients will walk through the door resulting in getting you out of the red and paying back loans in just a month or two. Each day the newness is wearing off, and Maggie comes in less and less. She has a family to raise, and that leaves you alone to figure things out. Maggie's husband calls you in two months asking you where all the clients are. He goes on to tell you that he does not have any more money to give you for bills and that you need to figure this out. All of the problems suddenly become "yours," and Maggie is nowhere to be found. You suddenly realize that you're in business with Maggie's husband, and, heck, you never really liked him anyway. Think long and hard before you go into business with your friends or family.

A partnership can work if it's with a fellow business person who is seasoned and understands the ups and downs of a business start-up. Maybe you're opening a women-only spin studio, and you decide to partner with a person who owns a yoga studio. Now that would be a great plan.

If capital funds instead of a business partner is the option you prefer, consider an investment Value Proposition. An IVP is the overall monetary value that an entrepreneur proposes that her company will deliver at some future point to the investor in exchange for the investor's money. The exchange amount the investor is looking for is a higher return on the investment. You must consult an attorney for this option and have an agreement designed.

Naming your business

Make it something easy for the consumer to understand. For example, if you call yourself "Hard Core Fitness," having fitness in the name will help the customer understand that it's a gym. On the flip side, the name Hard Core will not appeal to most women. Another idea is to use your community's name, for example "Huckleberry Fitness for Women." The best advice I can give you is to consult others and do a survey before choosing a name. I also suggest that you make your business's name different from your corporate name. Protect yourself, first and foremost, and speak with your accountant and attorney for advice.

Form an entity type (corporation, nonprofit corporation, or limited liability company ("LLC")). An accountant can advise you concerning tax issues, or an attorney can advise you concerning liability, taxes, and other issues. Do your homework. This is more important than a business name.

File with both your state and local community. Each state's requirements vary, so go to the Internet and pull up your state and local government's sites. Do it right the first time.

Apply for a Federal EIN or TIN. This is your awesome IRS tax paying number. The government has made it very easy for you to go online and apply. Please make sure that you're clicking on the government's site when doing this yourself, as your search will pull up many businesses that charge you to obtain this number. This is free and easy to apply for online on your own.

Once you have received your Tax ID, go to the bank and open an account!

Your bank account is opened! Now it's about to get exciting! If you have never rented a space before, I encourage you to hire a commercial real estate agent to guide you in your search. It's no cost to you. The landlord pays their commission. The real estate professional can guide you in negotiating the cost per foot, free months of rent, the length of the lease, repair coverage in case the AC/heater goes out, and much more. Do you know what triple nnn is? How about CAMS? If not, call a realtor before you begin your search! I have signed many leases. Please make sure your lease has these two important items:

1.) Have the landlord agree in writing to cover the mechanical components of the building such as the AC/heating/plumbing for the first 6 months of the lease. You have no idea how the previous renter treated those vital units. An A/C repair could knock you out of business your first year.

2.) Ask that your rent be due by the 10th of each month. If you bill your clients on the first of the month, those ten days give you room for all the revenue to come in. Pay your utilities and other expenses on the 15th of each month.

Now that you have the most awesome location, you need to turn on your utilities. Most utility companies require a deposit for a new service address. The deposit will be based on your credit, not the business. If the deposit is more than you can afford, go online and search for Utility

Bond Company. The cost of the bond will be a fraction of the full deposit, and you can keep your cash flow for more important initial investments.

Build your own web site with a web builder service or hire a professional. Your choice will depend on your budget. If you need to constantly update or add content, then a web site builder is a more affordable choice. You may be surprised at how easy it is to design your own website. Look around at your competition to get ideas. Remember that too much content will overwhelm viewers, so keep it simple. Be your best customer and make sure it has everything you're looking for when you shop.

Design a Logo

It is a much needed branding tool for your service/product. Sketch out your idea on paper. A logo can be a picture, your business name with a cool font, or a funky design. The sky is the limit. Be creative, but ask your friends and families their opinions before choosing the one that will be on your front door. Awesome sites like elance.com can be affordable ways to find someone to produce your new logo idea. They will send a .jpg file you can use for all your printing needs.

Purchasing equipment for a women's only studio can save you thousands of dollars. If you're starting a functional fitness facility, you will need barbells and weights. Everything is sold by the pound. Initially, you will purchase smaller women's grip bars and lighter bumpers. As your business grows and your ladies need to be challenged, you will make additional purchases for heavier weights and larger bars. It never makes sense to buy too much or to buy items that the average female will not be able to pick up and move when they initially start your program. If you're opening a Spin Studio, start with 15 bikes -- not 30 bikes. You're better off to offer more classes and fill up the 15 bikes every session instead of having empty bikes. The "less is more" approach works in this scenario. Clients want to be part of something that sells out, and the "less is more" approach works.

Signage is incredibly expensive. An illuminated sign on a building can cost between $2,000 - $3,000. I was blown away by my first quote for an 8-letter Pan Channel illuminated sign. The cost was $5,000. That price was not in my budget, but your landlord or building association expects you to have signage within 30 days of moving in. The clock starts ticking as soon as you sign a lease or buy a property. The landlord or property manager will provide you with the specs for the sign; and if you do not need an illuminated sign, your best bet is to go with a foam sign. They range in price from $600 - $1,500. Do your homework regarding signage before you sign a lease or purchase a building.

A client management system will become the first administrative assistant you hire. You must sign up and utilize a system in order to keep your clients and revenue organized. The systems on the market today allow you to take photos of each client, which is an awesome way to remember names and faces. They also help with attendance tracking, so you can send out e-mails if they miss class. And most importantly, they assist with revenue generation. Monthly billing using credit/debit cards or electronically drafting from checking accounts is the only way to run a business. Do you carry cash or checks anymore? I don't, and I am my BEST customer. Do your research and shop for a system that offers ease of use for you and your clients. If you plan on having clients reserve classes, make sure your system allows them to use their smart phones to reserve class times. Ease of use during your demo of the product should be your determining factor in your purchase of the product. In addition to the fee for the client management system (most are monthly and range from $75-$125), you will need to pay processing fees for your banking transactions. It is very important to be a smart shopper and not give away your revenues. Processing fees range from 2-3% of your transaction amount.

Hiring Staff

Think before you hire. First off, do you really think you can pull off being the only person running all the classes and the front desk? I don't recommend it. You need at least one additional coach to start. I understand this will cost money, but you will quickly find out that it takes money to make money. You better prioritize selling your service or product at first with the passion and desire you have to make this a successful business. It's a no brainer when I say that you and whoever you hire must be a certified trainer in your specialty. If you as the owner are not certified, how do you know what you are hiring for? How are you of service to your clients? So from here on out, I am going to assume you are certified in your trade and on top of your initial certification. I will also assume that you have 5-6 more certifications in additional activities such as USAW, kettle bells, endurance, spin, mobility, gymnastics, and the list goes on. Education is fun, and it will make you an expert with a high quality product/service that the public will demand. I want your employees to have the same or close to the same certifications as you do. Now you need to look at business budget and decide how much you can afford to pay someone. This should depend on their certifications, experience, and knowledge. The final step is finding employees. It's always awesome to be able to hire from within your fitness facility; but if you're new and just starting out with zero members, I suggest placing a Craigslist ad, newspaper ad, or ask friends and family who they recommend. When you find a new, have them sign a non-compete/employment agreement. Protect yourself from day one. I never like to think the worst of people, but you must protect your new business. And if the person you're hiring is not willing to sign it, then you definitely do not want them to be part of your team. Set payroll expectations and decide if a bonus structure will work for your budget. In my facility, I offer an intro class to new clients with a limited number of spaces that meets for 5 days. I pay the coach their normal hourly rate, and I give a $20 bonus for each person that joins the gym at the end of the 5 days. Make sure to set them up as employees and not contractors. Ask your accountant to help you with this tax issue.

I also encourage you to write an Operations Manual. It can be 5 pages or 20 pages, but it's the daily road map that you and your employees will follow.

Now let's open for business. It's time to get the word out. Did you call the newspaper and have that article written? How about the morning TV crew? Will they be attending a class? Were the flyers dropped door to door? Did you join the Chamber of Commerce?

Your sign is on the building, and a big WELCOME banner is installed. Your new employee is standing next to you, and no one is in the facility. Close the book and re-open it to the MEDITATION/AFFIRMATION section. Are you putting out positive vibes to the universe? Do you believe in your product/service? If so, and you're standing there with a smile on your face with all the hope and excitement, I guarantee you that people will start walking through your door. If you're standing there with a frown on your face saying, "this is not fair," and, "I don't understand why no one is here," negativity is rewarded with MORE negativity. No one will ever show up! Always remember your glass is half FULL!

Important things to remember:

Meditation, affirmations, and confidence are the KEYS to your SUCCESS! Be a giver and outwardly display happiness, and you will attract like-minded clients that want your products and services.

The WOMEN'S ONLY market will make $50 billion in revenue this year. Grab your piece of the success!

You are your own best client.

Write a handwritten thank you note each week to a client.

Building a strong happy COMMUNITY starts with you.

Be a constant student! I challenge you to read a book each month and listen to podcasts daily. You always need to be expanding your knowledge and your potential!

Ask for forgiveness, not permission. We all make mistakes and grow from them. Push the envelope and make things happen. Do not stand on the sideline.

Help your clients do what they are good at! If your community of women loves to run, have an endurance training group on weekends.

Most people choose unhappiness over instability. This journey is not for a person who craves financial security. Let's jump in together and open your dream business!

Women are forgiving, and understanding your client base will support and lift you up if you are honest and caring with each individual that walks through your door.

About the Author

RebeccaFerente.com and WomenintheGym.com both offer awesome mentoring programs with a variety of packages over the phone or in person. E-mail rebeferente@gmail.com for more details.

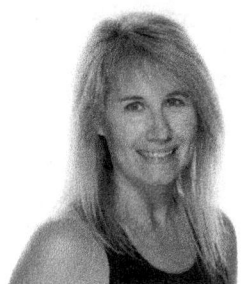

Rebecca Ferente, is a registered nurse, certified personal trainer, and has a bachelor's degree in business. She received her first fitness certification in 1999 and has continued to grow and expand her knowledge base. Rebecca currently holds certifications in CrossFit, Olympic lifting, kettle bell, gymnastics, mobility, endurance, spin, nutrition, as well as maintaining three additional personal trainer certifications.

She is a celebrity personal trainer and a nutrition specialist with a large fitness consulting business. Her most important job is being a wife and mother of four children and one grandchild.

Rebecca enjoys serving the female population, encouraging and helping women to get and stay well. Helping all fitness levels achieve confidence in nutrition and fitness are her top priorities.

www.WomenintheGym.com
www.RebeccaFerente.com

Rebecca's favorite quote:
"Sometimes you just have to stop worrying, wondering, and doubting. Have faith that things will work out, maybe not how you planned, but just how they're meant to be."

Find a mentor! You need a support system. Don't do this alone. Constructive criticism will make you a success! Start now by stepping out of your comfort zone and live your dreams.

Rebecca Ferente & Associates LLC is a world wide consulting company with offices in the US and Europe. We offer Business Consulting, Seminars, and Mentoring programs with a variety of packages over the phone or in person. E-mail rebeferente@gmail.com for more details.

25 "Butt Kickers" to make you Successful at LIFE!

1. Learn something new EVERYDAY.
2. Take a risk. I promise that you will grow from it.
3. Write 2 thank you notes per week and mail them.
4. Remove e-mail and Facebook from your cell phone.
5. Say please and thank you!
6. Respect your elders.
7. Work out every day.
8. Look people in the eye and shake their hands.
9. Smile when you answer the phone.
10. Say GOOD MORNING to a stranger.
11. Slow down!
12. Don't tell people that you're rich!
13. Turn off the news and find happy positive things to focus on. You and your friends will appreciate your vibes.
14. Do something that makes you uncomfortable.
15. Leave your phone behind and enjoy dinner and dates with family and friends.
16. Get out of debt! Pay credit card bills in full every month.
17. Clean out your closed every two months and de-clutter your home.
18. Don't SPEAK.........LISTEN!
19. Grab a real BOOK and read it.
20. Help a friend.
21. Be positive! When a negative thought comes to mind, tell yourself, "no thank you...go away!"
22. Laugh EVERYDAY!
23. Save money.
24. Tell your family you care.
25. Disconnect from the wireless world at least once a week.

New Business 3-Ring Binder Contents:

Business Registration Forms (LLC, Corp, etc.)

Tax Identification (IRS e-mail with your EIN)

Business Licenses (State & Local)

Bonds and Insurance (Equipment/Renters and most important --covering your clients' injuries)

Business Plan

Loan Documents (including credit cards)

Lease or Mortgage Paperwork for your space

Employee Work Contracts/Contractor Agreements

Staff 3-Ring Binder (visible brightly colored OPERATIONS Manual) You will need to update this regularly as procedures change.

On the inside cover, list IMPORTANT PHONE NUMBERS (for emergency, local hospital, fire, police, landlord, owner's phone)

Blank Injury Reports

Hours of Operation and Classes (Update regularly)

Pricing and Packages, Cancellations, Billing   (Update Regularly)

Staff List and Contact Phone Numbers

Computer Log-in passwords

Paper Client Waivers and New Client Info forms in case computer system is not working.

Daily Procedures (step by step): turning on and off lights, AC/Heating, throwing out trash, cleaning equipment, sweeping and mopping, anything and everything you would do when you come in first thing and when you close at the end of the day.

Must Haves for a Female-Only Fitness Facility

If you're opening a Functional Fitness Gym:
Wood or Plastic Dowels (do it yourself project)
Female Weightlifting Bars
Rubber Bumpers and Small Plates
Clips for barbells
Wall Balls 10#, 12#, 14#
Gymnastics Rings
Pull-Up Rig (you can build this yourself)
Pirouettes (you can build this yourself)
Jump Boxes for box jumps (you can build this yourself)
Kettle Bells 15#, 18#, 24#, 35#, 44#
Jump Ropes
Bands for pull ups and stretching
Climbing or Battle Ropes
Optional: Rowers and Stationary Bikes
AB Mats
Foam Rollers & Lacrosse Balls for stretching

If you're opening a Spin Studio:
Start with 15 bikes and a great online scheduling system.
More classes and smaller groups will cause a buzz.

Towels for clients to purchase
Moderately priced Sound-PA system

Best advice my fellow gym owner friends
have ever given me...

Form a relationship with all of your members. Greet them by their first name every time they walk through the door and keep a clean facility! Clean is so key! But don't expect time off -- especially at first.

Have everything in writing, and I mean everything (examples contracts, injuries (even ripped hands), waivers, deals, etc). Never be afraid to hire people better and smarter than you!

Never forget what it's really about -- changing the lives of your members for the better. Oh, and lots of toilet paper. Always over estimate!

Don't blur the line - it's easy to let it become almost too much of a community, and things can get too laid back, too relaxed. People will start to take advantage of your time and resources. I hope that doesn't sound harsh. We have a great community. We are going out on a float trip in a couple weeks, but there are certainly times when people cross the line in their expectations. And that's our fault for not making that line nice and bold from the get-go.

Keep your bathrooms clean, greet everyone by their first name, don't bang your clients (especially the married ones), charge more, don't be afraid, don't sell Advocare, send random postcards, celebrate the small things -- not just the top athletes, find the most popular girl in your town and get her in amazing shape - this will bring you THOUSANDS in revenue, train lots of hairdressers, don't be a douche, and finally -- love people.

Start out right. Use a scheduling system (one that integrates with your credit card processing is best), have a place for your athletes to log results, use auto-pay (preferably on the first, it keeps things easy), and make sure your web site looks good and is easy to read

Stay true to the reasons you opened. Don't worry about what other boxes are doing. Whatever you think your expenses will be....double it!

Treat it like a business, not a hobby. It can be fun and rewarding if done right or a real f'n grind if not taken seriously.

Don't pay attention to the #'s of members you hear people talking about. Pay attention to what you can control, not the BS.

#1 is understanding the work and time that is needed to put into a business. It's not always as glamorous at it looks from a member's perspective. Get a good accountant.

Fun signs to use in advertisements:

NO MORE!
EXCUSES!

A ONE HOUR
WORKOUT
IS 4%
OF YOUR DAY
no excuses

www.ingramcontent.com/pod-product-compliance
Lightning Source LLC
Chambersburg PA
CBHW070528290526
45790CB00003B/1348